This Notebook Belongs To:

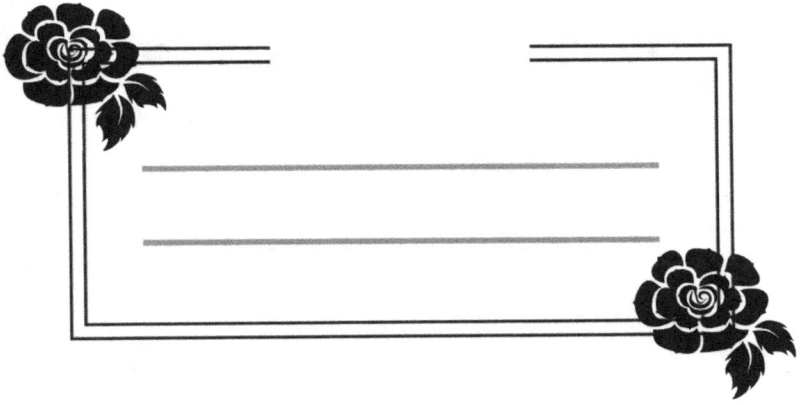

Enjoying this Notebook?

Please leave review because we would to hear your feedback, opinion and advice to create better products and service for you! Also, we want to know how you creatively use your notebooks and journals.

Thanks for your support!

You are greatly appreciated!

www.ingramcontent.com/pod-product-compliance
Lightning Source LLC
Chambersburg PA
CBHW070233220526
45465CB00004B/1416